EAT YOURSELF SLIMMER

Fat-Burner Foods & Recipe Book of Fat Burning Super food Smoothies with Super Food Smoothies for Weight Loss and Smoothies For Good Health

Dr. Anderson Brookes

Table of Contents

CHAPTER ONE

TOP FAT BURNERS FOR RAPID FAT LOSS

For the recently wellbeing cognizant, the choice to begin carrying on with a sound way of life can be overwhelming. While count calories and exercise are basic for sound living, there is more you can do. Fat terminators are a powerful supplement to consume fat and lift weight reduction. At the point when taken related to a solid eating routine and customary exercise, fat terminators can assume your weight reduction to the following level.

Picking the best fat eliminator can represent the moment of truth your weight reduction venture.

This book portrays a couple of compelling fat copying fixings and depicts how they work to assist you with losing undesirable weight.

It's critical to take note of that while fat killers are viable; they aren't a substitution for a sound eating regimen and exercise. They can't consume fat alone. So as to get results you'll have to eat a sound and adjusted eating routine and exercise normally.

ALL OUT DAILY ENERGY EXPENDITURE

A compelling method to gauge your advancement is through standard computations of your Total Daily Energy Expenditure

(TDEE), a gauge of your calories consumed every day. A TDEE adding machine will initially utilize your sex, age, weight, and tallness to figure your Basal Metabolic Rate (BMR). At that point, your BMR is increased by a movement factor.

Since an enormous piece of figuring TDEE is estimating your degree of physical movement, the computations might be powerful—and your advancement may be observable—when exercise is considered.

BASAL METABOLIC RATE

Your basal metabolic rate alludes to the measure of calories essential for your body to just play out it's vital capacities to keep your organs working. Figuring BMR doesn't consider any physical action on your part. In this way, it is basically what your body needs when you don't do anything. Henceforth, its substitute name, Resting Metabolic Rate (RMR).

Weight put on and weight reduction happen when the body expends pretty much calories than it needs, separately. At the point when you know your BMR, you can diminish your every day caloric admission as expected to get in shape.

Most of your weight reduction will originate from your eating routine. Bringing down your caloric admission is critical to consuming fat. In case you're attempting to shed pounds, a solid eating routine ought to be your top need. Exercise and fat terminators will give you an additional lift to shed your fat; however utilizing fat killers alone won't deliver any critical outcomes.

At the point when taken effectively, fat killers can help increment your BMR altogether. An ongoing report found that a solitary portion of a thermo genic fat misfortune supplement (fat eliminator) altogether expanded members' basal metabolic rate contrasted with benchmark estimations. The specialists likewise noticed that thermo genic enhancements may likewise help increment vitality use and fat oxidation without unfavorable impacts.

Fat eliminators increment the measure of calories your body consumes very still by advancing the procedures of thermo genesis (consuming calories to deliver heat) and lipolysis (separating lipids).

It is imperative to take note of that for ideal outcomes; fat terminators ought to be taken in the best possible doses to dodge unfavorable impacts. Continuously allude to the item names to locate the right measurements.

CHAPTER TWO

CALORIES AND MACRONUTRIENTS

Macronutrients (macros) are particles that give our body vitality. The three macros are fats, protein, and sugars. While they are found in all nourishments, the measure of each macronutrient crosswise over nourishment types contrast.

When following a weight reduction diet, checking calories and macros are similarly significant. While watching calories will assist you with realizing the amount to eat, watching macros will enable you to comprehend what to eat. For instance, expending 100 calories from a serving of cake and 100 calories from a banana won't affect your body? Utilize our calorie and large scale adding machine to discover customized suggestions that will assist you with hitting your weight reduction objectives.

There are 3 different ways to successfully get more fit:

1.   Increase your digestion

2.   Curb appetite longings

3.   Live a weight reduction way of life

The top fat eliminators talked about in this article contain fixings that work to build your digestion and check hunger desires. Whenever taken as prescribed with a fair diet, they will prompt a sound weight reduction way of life.

There are 6 fixings normally found in fat terminators, which are all sheltered and successful

1. GREEN TEA EXTRACT

Green tea separate contains an assortment of segments that help with boosting digestion. Conceivably the best of these is epigallocatechin gallate or EGCG. EGCG diminishes fat blend, builds the breakdown of fat, and amplifies your body's use of glucose.

Green tea likewise contains cancer prevention agents known as catechins. Catechins help with shutting out a chemical that assaults adrenaline and noradrenalin which are liable for moving fat stores and boosting your digestion. This is on the grounds that the higher your adrenaline and noradrenalin, the higher your pulse and internal heat level. Along these lines, your body consumes calories quicker.

As one of the most normal fat eliminators, green tea helps shed stomach fat misfortune to expand triglyceride levels.

2. CAFFEINE

Despite the fact that caffeine has an awful notoriety, caffeine anhydrous (the unadulterated type of caffeine) is a successful fat terminator. Caffeine attempts to consume fat in numerous manners.

To start with, caffeine helps your digestion. Truth be told, caffeine can support your caloric consume by as much as 150 kcal every day.

Caffeine likewise gives a jolt of energy which is especially valuable before an exercise. The more vitality you consume all through your exercise, the more fat you will lose.

At long last, caffeine diminishes the rate at which glucose is processed during a vigorous exercise. This implies your body will take more time to tire, and you will consume increasingly fat.

The drawback of utilizing caffeine as a fat terminator is that in the event that it is abused, your body will get acclimated with it and it will lose its viability. It is essential to take breaks each other week to accomplish ideal outcomes.

3. FORSKOLIN

While Forskolin is still generally new, introductory examinations show positive outcomes. In an examination posted by the National Center for Biotechnology Information, it was discovered that Forskolin caused "good changes in body structure by fundamentally diminishing muscle versus fat ratio" and expanding slender muscle.

The investigation additionally found that Forskolin expanded bone mass and testosterone levels in overweight men. This is critical in light of the fact that testosterone is significant in keeping up bulk, just as expanding your caloric consume.

4. 5-HTP

At the point when taken with Griffonia Simplicifolia, 5-HTP produces serotonin which has a few weight reduction related advantages. 5-HTP additionally diminishes hunger longings and along these lines lead to decreased weight and gut fat.

The International Journal of Obesity distributed an examination in which 27 overweight ladies were isolated haphazardly into two gatherings. The primary gathering was given

5-HTP characteristic plant removes, while the subsequent gathering was given a fake treatment. The examination indicated a critical increment in satiety of members who got 5-HTP over an 8-week time frame.

A few examinations have additionally indicated that 5-HTP helps in a roundabout way with weight reduction by expanding serotonin levels and melatonin generation. Expanded serotonin lessens the danger of tension and misery, which may prompt indulging. Expanded melatonin creation prompts a more beneficial rest plan, enabling your body to work appropriately.

5. L-TYROSINE

L-Tyrosine is an amino corrosive liable for making adrenaline and noradrenalin (which, as recently referenced, supports your digestion and moves fat stores). L-Tyrosine has been appeared to increment thermo genesis. Thermogenesis is the way toward consuming calories to create heat. Since thermo genesis consumes calories, it normally prompts weight reduction.

L-Tyrosine has likewise been known to connect with expanded dopamine, which lessens uneasiness and avoids weight gain.

In blend with the enhancement ephedra, l-tyrosine has been known to diminish hunger yearnings; however, l-tyrosine all alone doesn't appear to have this impact.

6. L-THEANINE

L-Theanine is additionally an amino corrosive and is normally found in green tea close by EGCG. Theanine will in general in a roundabout way advance weight reduction.

L-theanine brings down cortisol levels, which diminishes nervousness. Nervousness will in general lead to undesirable propensities, for example, gorging and a sleeping disorder. Gorging can be a major difficulty for somebody attempting to get in shape and lack of sleep likewise hinders the weight reduction process. By lessening tension, L-theanine can help individuals in maintaining a strategic distance from these undesirable practices and carrying on with a sound way of life.

CHAPTER THREE

GET FAST RESULTS

Every one of these fixings is just powerful when the three weight reduction techniques are in play (expanding your digestion, checking hunger yearnings, and carrying on with a weight reduction way of life). When appropriately applied to a sound eating regimen, noteworthy outcomes can be accomplished.

In case you're keen on shedding fat, look at our enhancements. Our fat killers utilize these fixings and more to assist you with looking and feel your best. With these fixings, you'll have all that you have to consume undesirable fat.

To remain committed to your weight reduction objectives, it's imperative to routinely compute your TDEE and eat an eating regimen containing your ideal calories and macros. The better you know your body, the more you can do to get it where it should be.

Normal nourishments and enhancements that consume fat

- Protein

- Polyphenols

- Caffeine

- Probiotics

- Green tea

- Fruit

- Preloading

- Fat-consuming pills

- Other approaches to shed pounds

- Summary

To shed pounds, an individual needs to consume a greater number of calories than they take in. Some characteristic fat eliminators, be that as it may, may enable the body to consume progressively fat by expanding digestion or lessening hunger.

To consume fat, an individual can't depend on a solitary nourishment or supplement. They additionally need to decrease their absolute calorie admission and increment physical movement levels.

Be that as it may, when part of an empowering diet and way of life, the correct fat terminators may assist speed with increasing weight reduction.

In this article, we talk about some potential common fat terminators and the proof supporting them. We will likewise cover fat-consuming pills, tips for utilizing normal fat killers, and other common approaches to get thinner.

Protein

Protein can bolster fat consuming and weight reduction from various perspectives. For instance, individuals who expend high-protein nourishments may feel fuller for more. Eating protein may likewise expand digestion, enabling the body to all the more proficiently consume fat.

Some high-protein nourishments contain fewer calories than high-starch food sources. For instance, an enormous bowl, or 124 grams (g), of cooked, plain spaghetti contains 196 calories and 7.19 g of protein Trusted Source. Conversely, two enormous hard-bubbled eggs contain 155 calories and 12.58 g of protein trusted Source.

A 2012 audit found that in the wake of getting more fit, expending a low-protein diet expands an individual's danger of recapturing body weight. To help weight reduction, numerous sources prescribe a day by day admission of 1–2 g of protein for every kilogram of body weight.

To boost weight reduction, an individual should attempt to pick lower-calorie proteins, for example, lean chicken, fish, and plant-based proteins. They should abstain from devouring exorbitant measures of red meat, singed nourishments, or food sources with included oil, fat, or spread.

Polyphenols are a gathering of synthetic compounds present in numerous nourishments, especially leafy foods. Some exploration proposes that polyphenol-rich nourishments may help weight reduction.

A recent report found that an eating routine rich in polyphenols may cooperate with microbes in the digestion tracts to help weight reduction, particularly when joined with an eating routine low in probiotics.

Different investigations of explicit polyphenol-rich nourishments, for example, curcumin, have likewise discovered a relationship with weight reduction. For example, a recent report found that taking curcumin supplements expanded weight reduction more than fake treatment in individuals who were overweight and had metabolic disorder.

A few nourishments that are rich in polyphenols include:

- apples

- pears

- grapefruits

- green tea

- turmeric

- spinach

- broccoli

- red wine

Caffeine

Caffeine is an energizer that can expand an individual's digestion. In any case, one 2018 examination recommends that caffeine may have a more critical impact on the body's digestion than analysts recently suspected.

The examination pursued 47 individuals from Finland who drank espresso however had quit drinking espresso for a month. The specialists found a relationship between espresso utilization and 115 metabolites.

When attempting to consume fat, it is ideal to pick low-calorie espresso choices by dodging unhealthy sugars, drains, and creams.

Probiotics

Probiotics are live microbes and yeast that are gainful to human wellbeing. Numerous nourishments contain probiotics, including yogurts and aged food sources, for example, kimchi, sauerkraut, and tempeh. Probiotics are additionally accessible as dietary enhancements.

The stomach related framework is home to trillions of microorganisms. Research Trusted Source proposes that expending probiotics can help improve the regular harmony among accommodating and hurtful microbes in the gut, just as help assimilation.

Some wellbeing specialists additionally guarantee that these gut-staying microbes may assume a job in digestion and weight reduction.

In any case, a 2015 precise survey found no information to help the thought that expending probiotics significantly affects weight reduction. The scientists inferred that more examinations are vital.

Green tea contains caffeine, which are substances that can energizer an individual's digestion. Green tea is likewise rich polyphenols.

A few examinations have discovered a little increment in weight reduction among individuals who routinely expend green tea.

In any case, a 2012 precise survey of past research found that this weight reduction was not measurably critical. The survey likewise found that green tea assumed no job in keeping up weight reduction.

Organic product

Sugar yearnings are a significant obstruction to weight reduction for some individuals. Controlling sugar yearnings with organic product may enable an individual to expend less calories.

Preloading

Some exploration recommends that preloading might be useful to individuals wishing to get in shape. Preloading includes expending a thick, low-calorie nourishment or drink before a fundamental supper with the goal that the individual feels fuller and eats less.

A recent report found that grown-ups with weight who preloaded with grapefruit, grapefruit squeeze, or water before dinners diminished their all out calorie consumption.

Fat-consuming pills

A few pills and enhancements guarantee to assist individuals with getting in shape. These pills fall into three classes:

Energizer pills contain caffeine and some of the time different energizers to accelerate digestion. They may assist individuals with losing some weight, however they can likewise cause quick pulse, hypertension, and different entanglements of over the top caffeine utilization.

CHAPTER FOUR

Dietary enhancements

Dietary enhancements incorporate fixings that may assist individuals with getting more fit. The viability of these fixings differs, and researchers have directed barely any examinations into these enhancements. Some contain polyphenol-rich nourishments or different fixings that may build digestion.

Endorsed weight reduction drugs

The United States Food and Drug Administration (FDA) have endorsed five professionally prescribed medications to help weight reduction:

- Orlistat (brand name Xenical) diminishes the measure of fat the body can assimilate. Orlistat is additionally accessible over the counter in a lower-portion structure called Alli.

- Lorcaserin (brand name Belviq) follows up on serotonin receptors in the mind to assist individuals with feeling fuller in the wake of eating.

- Qsymia is a mix of phentermine and topiramate. It works by diminishing craving and making individuals feel full more rapidly.

•   Contrave contains a mix of naltrexone and bupropion, which are drugs that specialists use to help treat dependence and sorrow.

•   Liraglutide (brand name Saxenda) may decrease sentiments of appetite and assist individuals with feeling fuller more rapidly. Specialists additionally use liraglutide to assist treat with composing 2 diabetes.

Weight reduction enhancements can cause genuine symptoms, so it is critical to converse with a specialist before utilizing them. Remedy weight reduction medications might be ok for certain individuals, yet they can likewise cause symptoms.

It is commonly best to attempt different choices, for example, making way of life and dietary changes, before considering weight reduction drugs. A specialist or dietitian can give counsel and backing to appropriate get-healthy plans.

CHAPTER FIVE

Tips for utilizing characteristic fat terminators

Characteristic fat terminators are not a substitute for customary ways to deal with weight reduction. Rather, they may assist individuals with consuming marginally more calories every day, consistently expanding weight reduction after some time.

To maximize regular fat terminators, it is ideal to incorporate them as a component of a reasonable, empowering diet. Try not to depend on them to consume fat alone or expect that eating nourishment will create moment results.

Consistently captivating in physical action is additionally a significant piece of any get-healthy plan.

Weight reduction is eventually the aftereffect of consuming a bigger number of calories than one devours. Decreasing day by day calorie consumption and accomplishing more exercise is the most ideal approach to get more fit normally. A specialist or dietician can give exhortation on appropriate health improvement plans and help individual set sensible objectives.

Basic approaches to fit more exercise into day by day life include:

•   taking regular breaks from sitting to walk or stretch for a couple of moments

•   using a standing work area

•   parking more distant away from goals to energize all the more strolling

•   walking or cycling to work

- taking up a game or physically dynamic leisure activity, for example, planting

Arranging suppers ahead of time can likewise help when attempting to adhere to an everyday calorie limit. Another tip is to consistently have a stockpile of restorative, low-calories tidbits to hand. These tidbits can assist control with wanting longings between dinners.

Rundown

There is no supernatural occurrence remedy for getting more fit. To get more fit, an individual needs to consume a larger number of calories than they devour. The most ideal approach to do this normally is by eating less and practicing more.

Notwithstanding, fusing certain nourishments or enhancements into a reasonable and invigorating eating regimen may help animate an individual's digestion and consume progressively fat normally.

THE END